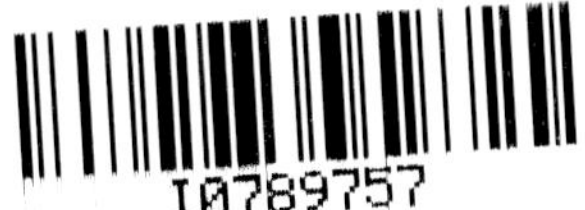


This Book Belongs To:

SALAD

SALAD

SALAD

SALAD

SALAD

SALAD

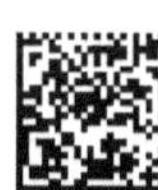
www.ingramcontent.com/pod-product-compliance
Lightning Source LLC
Chambersburg PA
CBHW070831260726
48654CB00025B/842

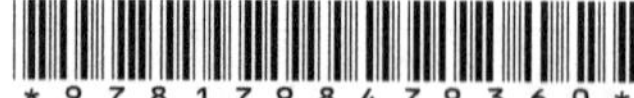